THE TOYBAG GUIDE TO

CLIPS AND CLAMPS

BY JACK RINELLA

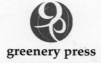

greenery press

Published in the United States by Greenery Press, 3403 Piedmont Ave. #301, Oakland, CA 94611, www.greenerypress.com.

ISBN 1-890159-57-3.

CONTENTS

DEDICATION

To Patrick – In appreciation
For countless clothespins endured

CHAPTER 1. AN INTRODUCTION

More than anything else, thoughts about clamps bring me back to images of my grandmother leaning over the railing of the back porch, her mouth full of clothespins, hanging laundry. If she only knew how I use clothespins now! It's the very fact that clothespins, and a wide variety of other clamping devices, are so accessible that makes them an ideal "pervertible." What toy comes 100 to the package and costs less than five dollars at your local grocery store? Grocery stores aren't the only local sources of clamps, either: pharmacies, hardware stores, and adult sex shops all carry a wide range of things that pinch and squeeze. Therein lies their pleasure.

Not only are clamps both easily available and affordable, the body parts where they can be applied are nearly too numerous to list: nipples, ears, lips, tongues, armpits, chests, arms, crotches and genitals, legs, feet, and fingers, to name the most obvious. The simple fact is that you can put clamps anywhere you can grab a bit of skin between your thumb and forefinger.

Since I first experienced clothespins as an aid to drying laundry, it wasn't until I attended a school for lower education at The Mineshaft, which was one of New York's most famous SM bars, that I first saw the real potential of those small wooden clips with the just-right metal spring. I remember being astonished when I saw a man whose top had stripped him naked, tied him spread-eagled on a St. Andrew's cross, and covered his body with clothespins. By the time the scene was nearly done, he was wearing more than 200 of them. It was then that I learned "Hey, I can use them for sadistic pleasure."

When I returned home, I took a half a dozen out of the laundry basket and added them to my traveling sex kit. I also used them on myself when I masturbated. It added a whole new dimension to my sex life.

In most cases clamps are harmless, leave no long-lasting marks, and offer a level of pain that is easily tolerated. The fact of the matter is that during most of their use, they feel painless or nearly so. There is a slight pain when the clamp is applied, depending upon its type, and then the body quickly grows accustomed to the device and the pain disappears.

Only by increasing the clamp's pressure or by twisting or hitting it does the pain return. On the other hand, removal of the clip, unlike the remainder of its use, can be quite painful, much worse in fact than any other stage in its application. The pain of removal can be increased by the simultaneous removal of many clamps at once (by stringing them in a line called a zipper) or by pulling them off rather than by releasing the spring or the screw.

Of course, any description of pain is going to be relative. What is nothing to one player might be overwhelming to another. What hurts in one place is hardly felt in another. For that reason, keep a good eye on your bottom's reaction so you can gauge what is really happening. Likewise, as I'll write again later, it's a good idea to try the toy on yourself so you know what it feels like.

Clothespins can be combined with other forms of entertainment. Some, who like to really get into it, for instance, will use a whip or flogger to remove them. The clips provide a great target and the whip insures that the clips' removal will not go by unnoticed. If you hit the wooden clips just right, the effect is quite dramatic as it causes them to almost explode off the body.

That observation does bring me to an important caveat. Clamps might go on really quietly and remain there with little or no obvious effect, but they often come off with great, if only momentary, anguish. For that reason, bondage is often a very important part of a clamping scene. Believe me, the pain of removal has turned more than one submissive into a screaming and swearing banshee. Better they be restrained than able to retaliate.

Needless to say, clamp aficionados have long gone past the use of simple wooden clothespins, though they certainly remain the mainstay of the fetish. Commercially available tit clamps range from those with smooth edges to those with teeth of varying size and number. Their tension or grip may be static or adjustable with the addition of a screw that can be used to open them wider, thereby reducing the pressure they exert. Other types rely on a sliding ring that rides up the shaft, intensifying the bite as it reaches nearer to the tip of the clamp.

Clamps come in all sizes and are made of a wide variety of materials, wood, metal, and plastic being the most popular, but many other substances may be part of an effective clamp. In the vendor area of a recent event I saw clamps decorated with rawhide, peacock feathers, paint, costume jewelry, and glitter. What the black-leather-and-denim-clad Old Guard would say about that is anyone's guess.

A recent visit to Mephistos Leather in Chicago proved that owner/partner/tailor Sheldon is a tit clamp expert. He showed me a wide range of clips and offered a surprising account of their origin. Many tit clamps, it seems, are simply adaptations of clips and clamps used by seamstresses and others who work with fabrics. The ones we call "Japanese," for instance, are actually used by workers who dye silk, and the needle-like tit clamps we call "pinchers" are used to pull elastic through the waistband of a garment. I thought tit-clamp lovers stayed up at night dreaming up new kinds of clamps, when in fact they where probably just raiding a local fabric store.

Clamping tools used by metal and wood craftsmen also serve well and are usually larger and therefore better used for clamping and pinching bigger parts of the anatomy, such as a wooden vise that might be used to squeeze a breast or a pair of testicles.

Before I continue, let me thank those readers who took the time to share their clamp stories with me. Throughout this book you'll read their quotes, giving real-life tales of the fun to be had with clamps. I would also like to give special recognition to Sheldon from Mephisto Leathers in Chicago for his excellent information.

With that introduction, join me in exploring the wide variety of clamps, applications, pleasures, and pains associated with that most accessible of SM toys – the clamp.

CHAPTER 2. A VIEW OF THE MARKET

If you have ever received a Lillian Vernon catalog, you know she would most likely gasp to know that her stainless steel bag clips have been perverted. I had to take some fine-grit sandpaper to the inside of each because of a slightly rough edge, but they hold up well when weights are added to them. I take great joy in knowing that she really does offer products to help this

HouseWife-Dom take care of daily "chores."[1]

There are two ways to consider the "market" for clamps: the first is the *what* and the second is the *where*. As the above quote makes clear, you can get a pervertible clamp almost anywhere. It only takes a little bit of imagination to spy a possibility and figure out that you can make it work.

The best method for determining a clamp's possible use is to first try it on yourself. The connecting skin between one's thumb and forefinger is the perfect place to do so. If you can handle the feeling there, then your bottom will tolerate it well in almost any other

---

1   *Diana, in an email sent on 06 Oct 2003. She also noted that you can find Lillian on-line at* www.lillianvernon.com.

place. This then leads me to the first rule of clamping:

Try it out on yourself first.

I write that because doing so gives you the only good understanding of how the clamp is going to feel. It is this understanding that allows you to use a specific clamp safely. I'll grant that there's not too much that can go wrong with the use of a suitable clamp, but that doesn't mean that all clamping devices are suitable.

The above idea about trying a clamp out on the webbing between your thumb and forefinger was taught to me more than twenty years ago. That doesn't mean that it's indisputable. A clamp is going to feel different based on where and how you attach it. Grab a little skin and it hurts worse, grab more and it may hurt less. Now look again, because I wrote *may* hurt less. Sensation is a varied event.

So let me remind you to try the clamp out on yourself in different places. Know your tools and use them well. Play in ignorance and reap the consequences.

What, then, makes a suitable clamp? It's one that stays in place, doesn't break the skin, and doesn't clamp so tightly as to crush the flesh underneath it. Some clamps might be unusable because they'll slide off, some because they pierce the skin and draw blood endangering the bottom through the possibility of infection, and some may actually pinch so tightly that they will injure the flesh.

Of course, most of the clamps we are considering are adjustable, so clamping "too tightly" is a relative term. Adjustable clamps only close too tightly if you screw them on too tightly. This is why trying the clamp on yourself is such a good idea. You'll know by experience how much you can close the clamp because you've felt the difference as the tension on the clamp is increased. No amount of looking or guessing is going to substitute for actual experience.

In most cases you can try the clamp on yourself even before you bring it home. There are some clamps sold in packages that can't be opened in the store, but I've found that most of the time there is at least some amount of pincher that is exposed so that I can give it the hand test. Quite frankly, most store clerks are too busy elsewhere to notice what you're doing. In shops that cater to us kinksters, it's obviously no problem if you do try them out. Just ask and you'll find the clerk is more than happy to let you experience the sensation, as this story demonstrates:

I have only just been introduced to these WONDERFUL little devices! I was staying at a gay resort in Florida and while killing some time I visited the leather shop on the premises and the clerk and I got into talking about clamps. A set caught my attention, I believe that he called them Japanese Cloverleaf clamps.

I asked him to tell me about them, and he said "Come here." He opened my shirt and placed one on each tit – YEOWWWW! In no time at all, my body adapted to them and I liked the way they looked and felt – WOOF. About that time some guys who were waiting for the bar to open up came strolling in. One particular guy pointed to me and brought his friends over to watch. The clerk told them that I was new to this and was showing me this set. The guys then started showing me other things about these clamps: when tension was applied to the chain between them they got tighter. After a short time with these four guys and the clerk applying various amounts of pressure to these

clamps and my tits, I began to de-
velop a slight sheen of sweat to
my body, which just added to the
whole experience.

After about an hour of our
"demonstration" and chat/play
the bar opened and I had to go
meet a friend for dinner. Before
they left, one of the guys came up
behind me and placed his arms
though mine bringing my arms up
behind my back, restricting them
and my movement. He then be-
gan to kiss my neck and ears and
suddenly one of the other guys,
with a smile on his lips, said "Well
if you like this, check this out!"
and suddenly removed them!!

OH MY GOD!!! I let out a
yelp and couldn't move and sud-

denly found another tongue down my throat. I thought I had died and gone to... Well, I would say heaven, but I don't remember ANYTHING about St. Peter and tit clamps!! They left with promises to see me later. I thanked the clerk for the learning experience with a promise to come back to make a purchase and then I left to find my friend, which I did.

We had to stop back by our room at the resort because I needed to change my shorts. It was my first orgasm without a single finger touching my cock. What a start to a Friday night![2]

---

2 *An email from PookieBear, received on 7 Oct 2003.*

I'll admit that not every foray into a store leads to an SM scene, but you get my point.

If the "where" of finding clamps is somewhat ubiquitous, the "what" is certainly more of the same. Relying on my friend Sheldon, I found hundreds of styles and sizes for all kinds of clamping scenes at my local leather store. Unlike the pervertibles from the grocer, these are manufactured just for us, with the disclaimer that they are "sold as novelties only." Styles vary from adjustable alligator, to nipple grippers, to tweezer clamps, battery clamps, macho clamps, tit presses, shark and piranha clamps, teasers, turn-ons, Japanese clovers, French clips, screamer tit clamps, gnat bites, hangman's nooses, tit-traps, clinging claws, micro pliers, sizzling sticks, and test tube clamps. (Different manufacturers and retailers may use different names, of course.)

What are the differences? Clamps come in all sizes and weights, made of metal, wood, plastic, and leather, biting and not, adjustable and not, padded and not. Let's look at that list again.

Clothespins. The simplest pervertible you'll find, these spring-loaded wooden and plastic gadgets work just right for a wide variety of scenes (figure 1).

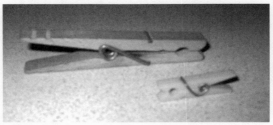

Fig 1. Clothespins come in all sizes, colors, and materials.

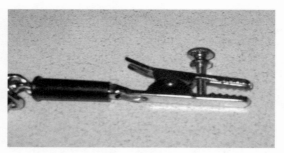

Fig 2. An alligator clip.

Adjustable alligator clamps. Probably the best known and most widely used of the clamping devices aside from clothespins, the alligator clamp is adjusted with a threaded screw and has teeth on its clamping edges. They are usually sold with the teeth covered with a removable soft vinyl pad. Two clamps, as are most of the clamps in this list, are usually joined by a chain (figure 2).

22

Nipple grippers are chrome cylinder clamps with smooth metal contacts and a tight squeeze. They are not adjustable.

Tweezer clamps and *sizzling sticks*, as their names suggest, give an adjustable pinpoint pressure. They are adjusted by the use of an o-ring that

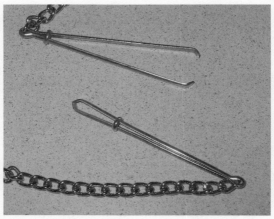

Fig 3. When you slide the ring on these pinches, they close their grip.

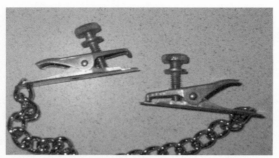

Fig 4. Note how the extra bite clamps into the flat surface on these macho clamps.

slides up and down the pincher bars. Originally called botkins, they are used in the sewing industry for threading elastic and turning fabric inside out. The tweezers have a slight tooth at the end, the sizzlers have vinyl knobs (figure 3).

Battery clamps have serrated edges and are tensioned by means of a non-adjustable spring. You can get these at a hardware store as well, but be warned that they have quite a bite and should only be used on advanced players.

Macho clamps have one edge that is flat and the other that bites with teeth. They are adjustable and usually wider and heavier than other clamps (figure 4).

Tit presses and *stocks* are small screw devices that clamp the body part between two flat adjustable crossbars.

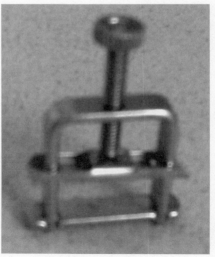

Fig 5. Tit press.

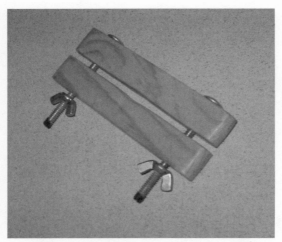

Fig. 6. This is another type of press, made of wood and big enough for squeezing nuts, a cock, or a tit. It is called a stock.

Tit presses have one screw, stocks have two (figures 5 & 6).

Man-eating, *shark* and *piranha clamps* are just what their names imply. The man-eaters are wide so that they can go around the tit to the meat behind it. The shark tit clamps have

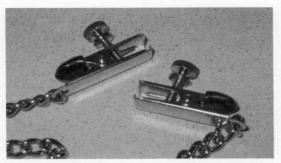
Fig 7. These man-eaters' wide claws are made to grab more meat.

jaw-like teeth while the piranha have rows of tiny teeth (figure 7).

Teasers offer padded protective inserts, mild pressure, and are "micro" in size.

Turn-ons are biting clamps that have an adjustable cylinder-shaped shaft. Turn the cylinder and the clamp bites harder. They are more elegant in appearance and usually a bit heavier (figure 8).

Tit locks close by squeezing and come in several sizes with adjustable pressure points.

Japanese clovers, originally used to hang silk to dry after it has been dyed, are popular devices, connected with a chain, with rubber contact points. Their uniqueness and popular-

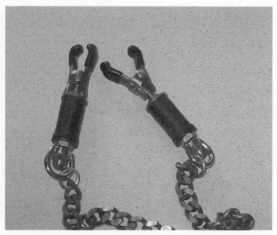

Fig 8. When you twist the knob on the lower end of this turn-on, you tighten and loosen its grip.

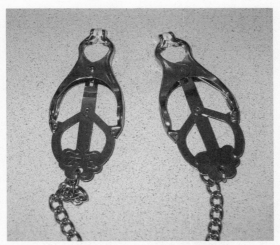

Fig 9. Japanese, cloverleaf, or butterfly — names vary, use does too.

ity arise from the fact that pulling on the chain makes the clamp bite harder (figure 9).

French clips are twisted (do we like that idea or what?) pieces of metal similar in appearance to paper clips. In fact, you can find them in stationery stores (figure 10).

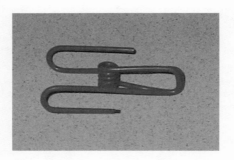

Fig 10. French clip.

Screamer tit clamps have an "over-bite" contact with a smooth, but very tight, surface. I think the name is self-explanatory.

Gnat bites are very small alligator clips, non-adjustable (figure 11).

Hangman's noose. Not exactly a clamp, this is a lariat of leather or string with a sliding clasp. Squeeze the fastener and pull the cord through it to make it tighter. They often come with hooks on the end of the cord for attaching weights.

Tit-traps are flat-surfaced springs. Push them to open.

Clinging claws are similar to tweezer clamps except that there are three or more prongs, closed with an o-ring.

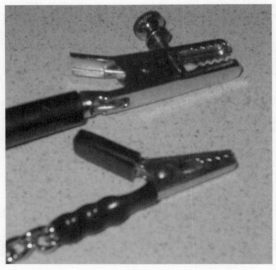

Fig 11. A gnat bite with its bigger sibling.

In spite of their appearance they are not extremely painful. Still, I advise you to try them on yourself first.

Micro pliers are smaller versions of vise-grip pliers, small enough to grab flesh, not so large as to be cumbersome. Check out the tool department of a hardware or electronics store for these.

Suction cups. If everyone who bought a snake bite kit used it for snake bites, there'd have to be a lot of snakes

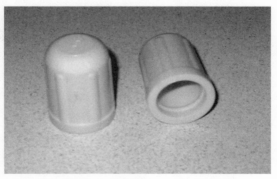

Fig 12. Suckers from a snake bite kit.

around, which of course there aren't. Also called "nipple suckers," these are used for play and are said to help increase the size of one's nipples. That's probably true, but it's not an overnight transformation (figure 12).

In all fairness, the above list only suggests the possibilities. There's no question that a sex shop is going to have all kinds of variations on the above themes. On the other hand you can find many of the above in hardware, craft, and sewing centers, except they most likely won't be connected by a chain.

Though we are considering clamps *per se*, the fact of the connecting chain is often a very desirable addition. Chains allow the addition of weights, facilitate contests, and enable the top to increase pressure by pulling. Consider this story:

I have a couple of suggestions to offer in regards to clamps. The first is a simple game a Dom played with me once: when he and I met, we both had a set each of clover clamps. I thought what he did was rather creative. He fastened one set from his left nip to my right, the other from his right nip to my left, then moved me about by moving his body back. Granted, clover clamps working the way they do, if I hesitated, we BOTH felt it, but it was an intriguing way to play for a bit.

Another thing I've gotten into is the electronic technician's friend: alligator clips! Granted, most alligator clips are a bit much for play, as the jagged teeth are too tight for many players. However, there are similar clips which I found at Radio Shack. So far, I've used them only on my own tits. The springs on them are strong enough that you don't want to leave them on very long, as local circulation becomes an issue. Still, they are INTENSE little buggers and fun to play with.[3]

One of the strong attractions to clamps is that most any small clamp-

---

3   *From LM in an email dated 7 Oct 2003.*

ing device can be perverted to our sadistic, pleasurable use. Just because I'm
writing about leather shops and hardware stores doesn't mean that a stroll
through almost any retail outlet will
turn up another gadget for the clamping sort of top, as these comments
demonstrate:

> *While browsing thru CVS (a*
> *pharmacy) one day, I happened*
> *to notice their selection of hair*
> *clips included big "banana*
> *clips." The guy behind the secu-*
> *rity camera must have gotten a*
> *chuckle as he watched me, for*
> *almost an hour, clamping hair*
> *clips to the inside of my arm test-*
> *ing their "bite." I found several*
> *that were acceptable and*

brought them home as a surprise for my slave.

As a subtle and prolonged torture, I had my slave lie on her back, spread-eagled on the bed. Her wrist cuffs were secured to her ankle cuffs by double clips. She was blindfolded and gagged. I had "Enya" playing softly in the background.

I chose a large, curved banana clip with a moderate bite and used it to clamp her entire pussy. The rounded plastic teeth gently bit into her from the perineum to her clitoris along the outside and securely at the base of her outer lips. Her reaction was immediate, both in body movement and a muffled *whimper. Once the clamp was in place, though, she realized it wasn't that bad and settled down.*

Next I took two smaller, albeit nastier, hair clips one third the length of the one on her pussy and placed them on her breasts, each one encompassing a nipple. The teeth on these two were sharper and made their presence felt much more acutely than the one on her nether region. These took her somewhat longer to adjust to but was (for me anyway) just as enjoyable to watch.

In a flash of inspiration, and since I was in a clamping mood anyway and noticing the effect the clamps were having, I de-

cided to add just one more.
From my bag, I retrieved several
clothespins and placed one, ever
so carefully, on the hood of her
clit. There was just enough room
left at the top of the banana
clip to take hold of the hood,
pull it up, and secure the clothespin around the shaft of the
clitoris.

It had taken perhaps ten
minutes to place all four clamps.
I knew I could safely leave them
on for about twenty minutes
since they really didn't cut off the
circulation, except perhaps for
the clothespin. So, for the next
ten minutes, I simply sat back
and enjoyed the show. I made
no sound and made no move-

ment except to light a cigarette. I was not disappointed.

The clamp on her pussy had already begun to work its magic and the ones on her nipples were beginning to dig in nicely. Even the least little bit of movement in her legs caused the clamp to embed itself deeper into the folds of her pussy lips. The twisting and turning of her upper body served to do the same to her nipples. There was nothing she could do to ease the insistent, ever-increasing bite of the clamps. Her juices began to flow. I noticed this and smiled to myself.

I watched the clock. I watched my slave. I knew precisely her level of excitement and debated leaving them on another five minutes. "It was early. Hell, we have all night," I thought. After twenty minutes, I started removing the clamps in the order I had placed them. First, I removed the banana clip and noted with some satisfaction the little red dots along the base of her lips. Her ass rose deliberately off the bed and I heard a sharp intake of air through her nose as I removed it.

Next, I slowly removed the clamps from her nipples. They had bitten so deeply into the soft areolae that little peaks rose with them as I pulled them off. They had bitten but not pierced the tender flesh. I'm sure, though, *that it must have felt as if needles had slowly been driven in. The sounds my slave made were exquisite music. The movement of her body told a story of pain, lust, and release.*

I took my time releasing the clothespin. I had five minutes to play with it. I gave it a flick of the finger just to watch her jump. I pulled it gently but inexorably upward and gave it a bit of a twist just to watch her squirm with delicious pain. I pushed the end of the clothespin slowly down in an arc, like a nail being pulled out by a claw hammer, till the tip of her clit, which had been standing straight up, was buried into itself. Then I let go and watched it pop back up. After releasing her clit, I did not touch her but rather let the body memory linger and fade of its own accord.

She was allowed to rest for five minutes before I put a clothespin on each nipple, and the two hair clips just above the line made by the banana clip. These were left on for twenty minutes as before and then removed. Her nipples, I might add, are pierced, so they are very sensitive to the slightest pressure. During each of her five minute rest periods I gave her a sip of water and one drag of my cigarette. Then we would begin again.

The banana clip was once more applied to her pussy lips. The twin hair clips were once again biting into the sensitive area around her nipples. And the clothespin was once more gripping her clit in a fond embrace. In all, this cycle of rotating clamps lasted two and a half hours. She had several small orgasms and I was learning a great deal about my slave.

Towards the end of that two and a half hours, I was suddenly struck with another bit of inspiration. We have a small "mini-vibrator" which is about two inches long and about a half inch in diameter. It only has one speed, "intense." I happened to notice that the space inside the large clip was just about right to hold this little demon, the head of the vibrator being just a bit bigger than the body so it wouldn't slip out. After clamping her clit, I dashed into the other room and brought back the vibrator and inserted it into the banana clip.

For the next ten minutes I watched my slave go through some of the most intense orgasms I had ever witnessed. Twice her hips bucked so hard she almost flung the vibrator from its holder. I heard her moans and cries build from soft mewling to gut wrenching screams and back again. Over *and over again she came until she had built a chain of orgasms a full ten minutes long. Then I released her.*

I removed the vibrator and the clamps and released the double clips holding her wrists to her ankles. I then put a pillow under her head and covered her with her robe. When she had regained her senses enough, I gave her sips of water. Afterwards we lay in each others arms, oblivious to the outside world and everything in it, completely lost in our love. This is but one of many such scenes.[4]

---

4   *Submitted by Mstrwicken on 7 Oct 2003.*

Chapter 3. Clothespins

For all the great variety available in clamping devices, there is no doubt that old-fashioned spring-loaded clothespins make a very popular toy. There are several reasons for this, not the least being their low cost. Besides price, though, they are easily obtained, need not be hidden, and pack just the right amount of pressure. Their tension is tolerable on most body parts, leaves neither scars nor long-term marks, and doesn't draw blood or spread infection.

I also have to admit to liking clothespins because they really are the lazy person's toy. Keep a bag by the bed and you won't ever have to get out of bed to get a toy. You can use them lying down while your partner stands or you can use them standing while your partner lies down. You can use a few or literally hundreds.

Though clothespins are generally consistent in tension, they do cause varying amounts of pain that depends upon their placement. The nipples, breast and chest, for instance, have one set of feelings when covered with clothespins, while the genital areas have another. If you haven't tried them nearly everywhere, then you haven't explored how totally versatile clothespins can be.

I once gave a clothespin demonstration at a bar in Detroit. A friend and play partner accompanied me, though he didn't act as the bottom for the scene.

The volunteer in Detroit ended up with 125 clothespins – and this was his first time! On the ride home, my friend asked me to do the scene with him, wanting me to make sure that I used more on him than I had in Detroit.

This is hardly a usual first scene. More realistically, simply start off with one or two clothespins. That, for some, may be more than enough. Put them on your bottom and notice the reaction. Wait a few minutes and take them off. See what reaction you get from that. Let your first time with clothespins (or your bottom's first time) be a slow and careful experiment. You can always go for more later, especially once you or they have experience.

You may then want to put them back on, perhaps in another place, perhaps not. You may get a great reaction and be encouraged to add more. On the other hand I certainly can't second-guess what's going to happen so you have to continually gauge the clamps' effects.

There are, to be sure, some areas where they just plan hurt like hell: lips, armpits, tongue, ears, and anus come to mind most readily. It is in areas such as these and at times when you're going to use more than a few that it's advisable to put your bottom into comfortable but secure bondage.

For all their initial mildness, clothespins, especially when used in great numbers, can cause some wicked pain. It is short-lived but in the moment of removal you're going hear some serious yelling and experience a good many gyrations on the bottom's part. For this reason bondage is actually a safety measure, because a flailing, screaming bottom can be a dangerous playmate, especially if by chance you've driven him or her to distraction and anger.

That comment leads me to rule number two:

> **When you're going to cause significant pain, use light bondage to protect your bottom and yourself.**

If I suspect the clamping scene is going to be either severe or of a longer duration, I usually begin by tying the bottom down with light restraint – I prefer spread-eagle, using leather cuffs on the wrists and ankles. Be sure that the restraints don't constrict nor hang too loosely. As with any bondage scene take care to check your bottom's hands and other extremities regularly to ensure proper circulation. You'll want to do most scenes with the bottom lying face-up on a mattress, though standing against a cross or a wall with eyebolts works well too. Even better is to put the bottom between two posts, so that you have maximum access to all body parts.

Any piece of skin that can be pinched between the thumb and the forefinger is fair game for the placement of a clothespin. In fact, the only area that I would say is definitely off-limits would be the eyelids, though there are other areas that you certainly would want to exercise care in clamping, as they are highly sensitive and the pain experienced may be much more than your bottom's limit at the moment.

Begin applying the clothespins wherever you like, though if you start in less sensitive areas, such as the chest, your bottom will last longer. I tend to put them on about ten at a time creating a symmetrical pattern on the body. First, one goes on each tit (assuming that the bottom does not have highly sensitive nipples), then I create a line of clothespins from one side of the chest to the other. Next I'll put a line of clothespins on the genitals.

Now's a good time to remind you about pain. It is going to vary from person to person, place to place, and from clamp to clamp. In spite of anything I write here, clamps can hurt and they can hurt like hell. Now they don't always hurt badly, but they can be full of surprises. Therefore, once again, watch carefully for reactions and remember that the pain is meant to provide pleasure, not an angry bottom who will never play with you again.

I usually take a short break between each set of ten while the bottom adjusts to what I've done, then begin applying more, perhaps on the scrotum or the arms. You can extend them in patterns from the crotch up the abdomen, down the legs and thighs, on the arms, neck, and armpits. Lastly you can put some on the mouth, the tongue, and the ears, though as I said they will soon hurt like hell on these more sensitive places.

Having gotten thus far, it's important to remember rule number three:

Clamps of any kind are going to hurt the most when, and during the minute or two after, they come off.

Once on, you can play with the clothespins by twisting or pulling on them. Be careful to gauge your bottom's tolerance level by watching his or her body language. More importantly, remember that even if the bottom seems to be tolerating the pain well, there is the possibility that they are toughing out a scene that isn't at all pleasant for them. Step back from what you're doing every once in a while (five to seven minutes) and inspect your handiwork, especially looking for signs of stress and fatigue. It doesn't hurt to simply ask how things are going as well.

Most commercial tit clamps come with a protective vinyl covering over the teeth, which can be easily removed to increase the clamp's aggressiveness. Be careful to save the protectors, as they are easily lost. Be aware that the vinyl tends to slide off a piece of flesh that has become sweaty or oily. The application of a small bit of cornstarch on the skin will absorb the moisture and make the vinyl stay in place. It doesn't take much starch, so be careful not to overdo it.

There isn't any really good way to take clamps off painlessly. *In any case,* the clothespins will hurt most when they come off, but by opening them rather than just pulling them off, you can mitigate much of the pain. Taking them off quickly is also an effective way to get it over with. Doing so slowly, one at a time is, of course, just more sadistic.

You can also mitigate the pain by providing a distraction. My friend Janet suggests, for instance, that a pleasant stroking, as with a piece of soft fur, near the clothespin as you take it off will make doing so much easier. This idea is a good one unless you're like me and would really hurt your bottom. Only you and your bottom know what kind of pain and at what level is satisfactory.

I asked Patrick, who sometimes has to take them off of himself, about the pain of removal. He said that taking two off at a time from different parts of the body seems to lessen the pain, as each pain cancels out the feeling of the

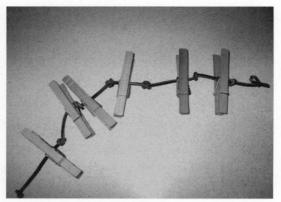

A short piece of rawhide is used to string a line of clothespins together. These are spaced rather far apart but will do the job.

other. Taking a single clothespin off very, very slowly allows the blood to seep back to the pinched area more slowly in a less shocking way as well. Certainly ripping them off hurts the most, which naturally leads to the creation of what is called a "zipper."

A zipper is a length of leather thong, cord or string that holds a number of clothespins together and is tied much like a string of pearls. They are often strung together with a small space or a bead between each clothespin, in lengths of fifteen to twenty-five clothespins each. You can certainly string fewer or more together – the actual number is determined more by one's degree of sadism and masochism than by any arbitrary yardstick.

Master and I use clamps in our play together. At first he bought two 96-count packages of Martha Stewart brand clothespins from K-mart and some twine and pony beads. We had a session of time together where I strung the clothespins in a varied amount of lengths or counts. Some strands were of six clothespins, some of 12 count, and some of 24 count. You probably know them as zippers. He placed them on the fleshy parts of my body and then ripped them off. Since I'm a masochist it was quite a rush.[5]

Another bondage/clothespin combination is to use the clothespins (or any clamps for that matter) as places to attach leather thongs or cords to your bottom. Pulling these cords tight, I often attach the other ends to the post of the bed or to eyehooks that might be available on a cross, the walls, or the ceiling. Alternately I will loop a string from a clothespin on one body part through an eyebolt or protrusion above

---

5   *Jorah Reign via email on 09 Oct 2003.*

the bottom and back to another clothes-pin. This means that movement in one part of the body is going to cause stress on another clothespinned part of the body.

In a previous quote we learned of a top who sat and watched the bottom's reaction. Alternately one can soothingly stroke the bottom causing sweet sensations to mix with the spicy ones. The stroking doesn't need to be limited to fingers either. Kiss, rub with your feet, suck, bite, and generally wiggle the clamps and the area around them.

Clothespins can be used in fewer numbers effectively as well. Try having your bottom wear a few during inter-course or put one on the lips of the mouth or the tongue while she performs oral sex on you. I like the feeling of clothespins attached to the bottom's nipples while he or she lies with their face in my crotch giving me head. I can then use my thighs and knees to push the clothespins into his or her flesh. It certainly motivates them to do a good job.

As said before, you can string two people together, tit to tits for a pulling game or a tug of war. There are almost no limits when it comes to ways to be creative with clothespins:

> *I wanted to tell you about a game some of us play around here in North Carolina, the colored clothespin game. I have no idea if other people do this.* [They most certainly do.] *The bottom is bound and blind-*

folded, but not gagged, and his scrotum is mostly covered with cheap plastic clothespins in various colors; i.e. red, green, blue, white. Leave a little space for more pins. Then the top chooses a clothespin, wiggles it, and asks the bottom what color it is. If he guesses correctly, it comes off. If he guess wrong, another clothespin is added. Like the game "Memory" or "Concentration," if the bottom is good, he can keep track of which colors he has called on a particular clothespin and get down to just a few. But the problem is that the pain starts to get to him and he gets frustrated and *forgets. The calmest bottom can do it, though!*[6]

---

6   *Written by Mistress Tempest via email on 8 Oct. 03.*

CHAPTER 4. PAIN MANAGEMENT

Though most of us wouldn't rate clothespins very high on the pain-induction scale, there are times when they hurt like hell. Likewise there are clamps and clips that plainly hurt without qualification. The pain that we consensual sadists inflict and willing masochists desire is the kind that leads to pleasure, as describe by Mstrwicken as "a chain of orgasms ten minutes long."

Differentiating between the pain that pleases and the injury that hurts is a crucial element in healthy BDSM.

Ensuring that what we do is pleasure and not harm is the responsibility of both partners. I've already suggested a couple of tactics to create a good clamp scene, the first being bondage and the second attention to the bottom's safety.

I can't emphasize too strongly that both the top and the bottom are mutually responsible in ensuring that all goes well. Neither can abrogate their responsibilities to act safely, sanely, and consensually. It's necessary, then, for the top to continually gauge the bottom's reaction, maintaining close awareness of his or her comfort level, circulation and breathing, pain tolerance, and pleasure.

Likewise bottoms must be certain that they are communicating the true reality of the scene to their tops. Toughing it out may sound like the way to go but it is a formula for injury. No degree of submission, masochism, or slavery entitles a bottom to remain silent in the face of physical harm. If your top is obviously unaware of what's really happening, then it's your duty to give him or her a very obvious indication of that reality.

Short of ending a scene, there are quite a few pain management techniques that will indeed allow any number of clips, clamps, and clothespins to create a great amount of pleasure. Remember in all of this, rule number four:

We do what we do for the fun of it. If it's not pleasurable or doesn't lead to pleasure, then don't do it.

That's not to say that there won't be pain. We sadists inflict pain for the pleasure we receive by doing so. We masochists accept pain as the route, the way to pleasure. We know that a certain kind of physical pain will be transformed into pleasure, if we but make it over that necessary threshold when the endorphins take effect.

In this process it is important for the top to understand what's happening. Our bodies adjust to pain incrementally, therefore the incremental application of pain (remember ten clothespins at a time) is an important technique, even if the number isn't. The breaks, the time-outs, and the pauses are all methodologies that allow the bottom's body to transform pain into pleasure. If you re-read Mastrwicken's story with that in mind, you will easily see that a three-hour session happened twenty minutes at a time. There were breaks for sips of water and even a puff on a cigarette! The clamps went on and came off and went on again. The scene had an easy, relaxed pace, with soothing music and a blindfold to reduce distractions.

In other scenes it may be necessary for the top to coach the bottom, reminding him or her to relax, to breathe, or to visualize the pain dissipating. On more than one occasion I've had to tell a bottom "It's OK, I'm taking them off" or "You can handle it, if you breathe deeply and relax." It's not that bottoms don't know these things, as many of them do. Still, a gentle reminder doesn't hurt.

Telling a bottom what is going to happen can often make the scene go more easily as well. For instance, you might say that there will be five more, and have the bottom count them. Knowing that there is a time when there will be no more (at least for the moment) makes taking the next one easier.

My slave Patrick, for instance, hates to have clothespins on his foreskin. It has long been an area that I have had to avoid. Wanting to get over that limit, pushy bastard that I am, I told him that he needed training in this area – foreskin training. When he agreed to the training, I put a clothespin on him and told him to relax. When that was accomplished, then I could move to clothespins number two, three, and four.

I had to watch carefully for negative reactions and talk him through it the first several times while I "trained" him. Now that he's used to it, we've moved on to lip training and ear training. God, I love being a sadist.

There are times, too, when there's more going on than just clamps. I remember a scene that happened more than a dozen years ago. I had been dating Stan for about ten weeks. He learned what he could endure and how to enjoy it. It was a mutually fulfilling time of training and affection. Stan was becoming a leatherman.

On the "night of the clothespins," he was kneeling buck naked next to my bed. His hands were tied behind his back. I looked into his eyes and over the next five minutes or so, I put twelve clothespins on his cock and ball sac, one by one.

I don't remember what, if anything, we were talking about. I do remember being my typical demanding self. I wanted to take Stan a bit further tonight, past a limit, into new territory. There was an intense feeling between us, though I have to admit I wasn't reading the scene as well as I thought.

Stan was taking everything surprisingly well. For a 21-year-old novice he was doing fine. At least that's what I thought.

When I put on the twelfth clothespin, Stan lost his temper and told me to stop, to take the clothespins off. He didn't want any more of this. Of course, I did as he asked.

I ended the scene right then and there but I wouldn't let Stan go home immediately. I convinced him to take a few minutes to talk things out. As we did, the real story came out.

For it wasn't the clothespins that had triggered his reaction. In the pain and intensity of the moment he had flashed on images of his childhood. I was no longer a leather top. Instead he saw his father, demanding perfection, pushing him to take it. It was an unpleasant experience and one at which Stan had often and repeatedly rebelled. He didn't so much want to me to stop as he wanted the Dad of his childhood to stop. The clothespins and I had pushed him into an emotional and psychological area that was hidden and long suppressed. The scene was a trigger for its release and revelation.

Experiences with depth, emotional release, and the gaining of insight are side-benefits of intense physical activity. Though we often forget, the many aspects of our lives are intricately woven together. Emotion affects thought which affects body which affects action and reaction. Each aspect of ourselves builds and feeds the others. Each "part" of us only seems to be a part. In reality we are one and complete in many dimensions.

So if you think it's the clothespins, or the leather, or the kissing, remember it's not the clothespins. What is it? It's the life experiences that we bring to the moment, the fleeting experiences that add up to life.

Chapter 5. Advanced Clamping

Though it really only takes a few clothespins to increase your pleasure, there's no doubt that more complex scenes can be thrilling. I've already touched on some of the ideas that I'd like to expand upon in this chapter. Zipper play can be enlarged into net play. Simple games can be made more complex. Bondage and clamping can be combined and weights added.

As you might well suspect, advanced play demands preparation, increased attention to matters of safety, and a very willing masochist. There's no time like the present to give you rule number five:

Be prepared for anything, because prevention is the best of all cures.

For most advanced clamp work you'll want to make sure that your bottom is well-bound and comfortable. Many times scenes are ended early because of some discomfort that could have been easily avoided by paying attention to the necessary details, so take care to start your play well, in order to get the most out of it.

I want to emphasize the importance of comfort in the last paragraph. If your bottom becomes cold, if circulation is cut off, if they simply become tired because you have them in an awkward position, then your pleasure and theirs is going to be at least interrupted and at worst the scene will end. Yes, we want to inflict pain, but the result of that pain should be mutual pleasure, not a bottom who ends the scene in disgust at the top's incompetence.

Good preparation means that you have all the equipment easily accessible before you begin your play – and that includes emergency equipment, such as a good pair of surgical scissors and a pair of pliers for emergency removal of ropes and chains. It also means that you have taken the environment into consideration. Having the lights at the right intensity, the temperature at a tolerable level, privacy assured, and distractions minimized are all part of good planning.

Since this book isn't, and can't be, a complete introduction to BDSM, I have omitted any discussion of finding a suitable partner and negotiating a consensual scene. That is not to imply that any use of clamps and clips need not to be mutually agreed upon. If you hope to experience any of these "advanced" scenes, consent is even more necessary. I'm not talking about assumptions, expectations, or innuendos here. Be clear with your partner about what you both want and enjoy. Prior agreement is part of good preparation. No one likes surprises.

If stringing your clothespins in zippers increases the pain threshold some ten times, then creating a net becomes the granddaddy of clothespin pain. There are several types of nets that one can use: a simple make-your-own of strong twine, commercial fishing netting, or material that is net-like. The procedure is to cover part or all of the bottom with some kind of mesh-like fabric and then attach the clothespins over the mesh onto the skin. There's no rocket science here, except be warned that grabbing a corner of the material after some fifty or a hundred clothespins are attached to it, and pulling it off your bottom is going to rip the mesh, clothespins and all, right off with an amazing burst of pain.

This is what "Loop Daddy" has to say about the net scene:

> *My favorite is a slight variation on the classic fishnet and clothespins. I tie my boy to a floating bondage table hung from chains. I hood him, cover him with a fishnet, and outline his body with clothespins attached to him and the fishnet. I*

put them down both sides of his body, inside his thighs, on both sides of his arms, nipple to nipple and a dozen or more on his scrotum. Sometimes I add a couple hundred more, but the outline is the important part.

Then I attach hooks or rope from the net to the chains supporting the table, use his always hard dick as a handle, and start moving the table. As I pull on his dick, the ropes attached to the chains pull and tug in every direction, making wonderful squeals of pain burst out of him. Moving the table in big circles is my favorite, because the boy begins to find a regular pattern and starts to know how to

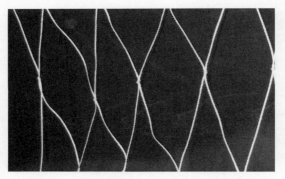

This is a photo of home-made netting. I simply bought some strong twine, cut it into seven foot lengths, and tied the pieces together. Granted, I'll never make a great fisherman, but it works in the bedroom.

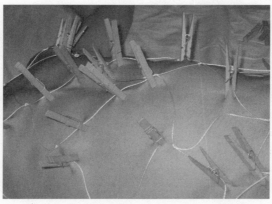

When pulled off, these clothespins will cause quite a yell. Music to a sadist's ears.

handle the pain. Then I suddenly change the pattern, which makes everything new and surprising again.

Eventually, I gather the ropes together and pull the fishnet and all of the pins off in one wonderful burst of agony for him. The last time I did this he came at that moment. A great thrill for both of us.[7]

Netting, as noted in Loop Daddy's quote, leads itself into the next degree of clamping – that is, the addition of twine, string, thongs, or cords. Secure your bottom beneath or near a number of places where you can attach cords

---

7   *From Loop Daddy in an email dated 10 Oct 2003.*

above him or her and you give a whole new meaning to the word "bondage."

There are many variations on this theme. You can use chains on the side of a bed, eyehooks over the bed or on the cross itself. You can have your bottom lie on the floor and use a chair on each side of them to fasten your cords or position them near a door that has a hanger on it. The idea here is to scout out your venue and be creative in finding places that will work for you. In any case, of course, be sure that the tether you use is substantial enough to hold the tension and the weight. A screaming bottom can pull a lot more than you think and you don't want to bring it all down around the both of you nonconsensually.

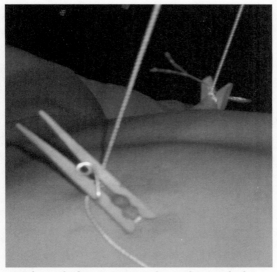

These clothespins are tied together, with the string looped over the top of a four-poster bed. The string is actually tied around the nipple. When the clothespin is removed the string slips right off.

Having found the right tethering points, you can either string from clothespin to tether or from clothespins on one part of the body to the tether and then continue to another part of the body, so that movement on one part of the body will exact its price on another. Similarly, you can attach the cord from one clothespin directly to another, as from a tit to a toe. When the bottom moves his or her foot, it's immediately felt in the tit.

Now that we've attached cords in appropriate places there's no reason, if

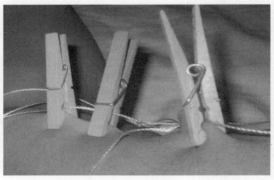

This picture shows a different way to combine string and clothespins. Note how the clothespins go over the string onto the flesh.

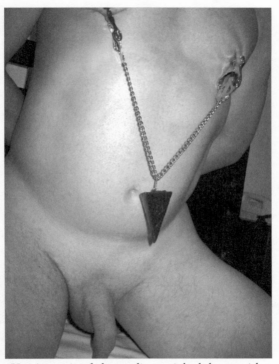

Here's a pair of clover clips weighed down with a fishing weight. Good for bottom-feeding bottoms.

you've done your homework, not to suspend weights from the cords. This is done most easily when the bottom is standing, but that is not a requirement. I have a four-poster bed. I attach a pair of alligator clips to Patrick's tits, a piece of cord to the connecting chain and throw the cord over the top of the bed. A light weight on the free end finishes the project.

By incrementally increasing the size of the weights you'll find that you can add a good deal of weight. Once again, watch the reaction you're getting from your bottom and play accordingly. Even the addition of small weights will have a desirable effect. Weights can be purchased at hardware stores, bait shops, and at secondhand stores. Alternately, you don't even need to use weights.

Heavier clamps, boots, and tools all make good weights. Avoid using things that are breakable or sharp.

As Loop Daddy wrote: "My other favorite tit toy is a pair of small (4-inch) vise grips which are infinitely adjustable, weigh a fair amount, and look great hanging from a boy's tits."

Remember in all of this that time is an important factor. Clamps are relatively harmless in the short term but the extended wearing of clamps may pose a danger. Therefore stay aware, check for circulation and numbness often, and move and remove the clips and clamps as necessary.

Playfulness is an important asset in clamp play, as amply demonstrated by the number of games you can devise with a few clothespins and a blindfolded bottom. Simple counting games or the "What color is this clip" are just two of the varieties on the theme. The color trick was described in chapter three. A counting game is just that.

Have the bottom count, either aloud or to himself the number of clothespins that go on and come off. By adding and subtracting quickly enough you can get him (or her) pretty confused and then "punish" them with the addition of more clothespins. Much of the fun here is psychological and a test of wits.

Marie writes an interesting story about games:

> *I very much enjoy the use of clamps during play. I will share two scenes that were fun for me. The best mind fuck*

ever done to me was a zipper on my labia. As I lay there assimilating the pain, I was ordered to count backwards from five. A simple task, yet I was frozen knowing that the end result would be ripping off my lower lips. My mind went blank; I couldn't even formulate the numbers, much less say them. The top sternly ordered me to count a couple of times; then apparently in frustration at my disobedience, said "Fuck it" and yanked the string holding the zipper. I literally levitated off the table in fear, only to find out that he had not interlaced the string with the clothespins. The good news is

I am still intact; the bad news is that mind fuck only works once.

On the top side, I enjoy attaching nipple clamps to toe clamps and having the bottom crawl as I spank, beat or otherwise torture them. It is also fun to form a train, where the clamps attach the scrotum of the first bottom to the nipples of the second as they crawl around, under strict orders to avoid distractions all the while providing many opportunities for distraction. Ahh, clothespins![8]

---

8   *Sent to me by LadyMynx4u in an email dated 3 Nov 2003.*

Not all clamping scenes need be stationary, either. You may want to send your clothespin-laden bottom into the kitchen to get you a glass of water. Just knowing that every step causes a sensation is worth the wait. You might send them crawling somewhere with a dozen clothespins on their genitals or have them do housework while wearing weighted tit clamps. This leads to the natural use of a leash or a pony halter or bridle. One step further and you can use a crop to make sure they move just right.

Taking this variation another step forward, pairing bottoms with matching clothespins and clamps can be fun too, or you can, as previously mentioned, clamp them to yourself. Crawling while decorated with clamps and cords can make a good parade too, but a single bottom will do if that's all you have available.

The more adventuresome sadist may want to use the crop just mentioned to tickle the bottom or, better yet, to tickle the clamps. Now the clothespins won't laugh, and your bottom might not either, but it will put a grin on a sadist's face. You can see why I suggested that the pain levels here be pre-negotiated. As we move into more intensity it remains important to make sure that all is consensual.

It's not the purview of this book to discuss whipping techniques, but experienced floggers, whippers, and caners may want to try to use their equipment to remove the clothespins. Don't try that unless you have experience with the implements just listed. Likewise, as any experienced sadist should know, be certain that your bottom has the experience level and willingness necessary to take such pain.

The secret in all of this is to explore and experiment. With endless possibilities I can only point you in the right direction to fully enjoy your body and that of your partner's. Following the rules I've mentioned in these chapters, there's no one way to do it right. Be creative, be imaginative, and be safe.

Mostly, though, remember to have fun, which is the best reason to clamp down on someone in the first place.

Appendix: An End Note About Tits

Tit play is an acquired enjoyment. By that I mean that many people don't know how erotic it is to have their nipples played with, but after a few sessions they learn that it is great fun and excruciating pleasure.

Perhaps some people have naturally eroticized tits – I'm told this is the case for many women. But for most men, I think, it just takes practice before we learn that we can enjoy our tits. I'm not sure there is a "schedule" *per se*, but simply that regular tit play will do the trick. Get yourself a couple of clothes-pins, a snake bite kit, and various kinds of tit clamps and use them on yourself or have your top use them on you. It's as easy as that.

At least it was as easy as that for me. Remember that I'm a guy. Women are going to have different experiences and other guys may react differently than me. We come in all shapes and sizes and have all sorts of different levels of pain tolerance.

One female friend noted that "my nipples were sexually pretty non-responsive until I nursed my kids, and have been extremely sexually responsive since then." She guessed this was the female version of the process I described above! She also wanted me to warn you that on many women, the nipples are not a "less sensitive area." The warning means that you have to know what you're doing and see how it goes. A clamp in the wrong place, after all, isn't fun if your bottom doesn't enjoy it.

On the other hand, if you're simply sadistic, no matter what I write about being cautious may not be the scene you want. In any case, negotiate it first, as doing so later may not be possible.

Buy adjustable tension clamps so that you can begin with an easy pressure and tighten them as your training session continues. A little tightening every once in a while will do amazing things.

The temptation, of course, is to take them off too soon. If you succumb, just wait a few minutes and put them back on. Start slowly and easily and build up to higher pressures and more pain. If they hurt too much, you are going too quickly.

Avoid cutting and tearing your tits, as this can lead to infection. If they are too sore or if they bleed, stop and give them several days' rest. Time to heal is important as the healing will build scar tissue and increase both your tolerance and your pleasure. If your tits are pierced you may try taking out the rings to see if that makes playing easier. Be careful, too, to avoid pinching the skin between the clamp and the jewelry.

It's helpful to remember that not all pleasure comes from pain either. It is important to vary the intensity of pressure. Light gentle touches and strong pinches both have their places in good tit work.

Common wisdom – generally unspoken – is that sex comes naturally and what you have and how you use it is what you're stuck with. There's no thought that sex can be taught or learned, but this wisdom is falacious.

Face it. We build our muscles and develop our minds. There are schools for dance, music, and architecture. There are gyms and football camps, coaches, instructors, and teachers of all sorts, but we leave sex to be learned on the fly, without any expert supervision, and the job is seldom done well. Other cultures teach sex in various ways but we Americans shy away from it. Sad to say, the majority of us learn it poorly, struggle with it often, and long for a better way.

I always thought that my tits were just my tits and useless since I am a male. I had no idea what they were for and didn't think they would ever amount to much. I was wrong. The nipples on a man's chest can be the source of an immense amount of pleasure. That much I've learned. Emails and conversations with my female friends give ample proof that their nipples can be fonts of pleasure as well.

A night in a bar where men expose their chests demonstrates that tits come in all shapes and sizes. What you don't see is that the variations can be developed. With playful attention, my own tits have grown in size and as they've done so, they become a greater source of pleasure.

I remember my first forays into tit work. Barely out in the leather scene, I'd put a clothespin on each nipple just to see what would happen. Invariably, I'd soon take them off. It was all pain. Well, almost all pain – hidden in the torture was a heightened sense of arousal and a bit of pleasure.

With practice I could take the clothespins, and then tit clamps, for longer periods of time. And with practice the pain diminished and the pleasure increased. The idea that an aspect of sexuality can be developed, actually learned, is important. It points us to a way of being, a way of looking at things, that affords us greater possibilities.

Yes, we may think that we lack sensitivity in our chest. Yes, we may shun partners who squeeze our nipples, but the truth is that many of us can learn not just to tolerate such activity, but actually to enjoy it. On many an occasion my tits have ached with a warm glow, both of pleasure and pain.

Playing with someone else's tits is another sensation. The pleasure is in the control and in the giving of pleasure. I see my partner squirm, writhe, as I use his nipples to dominate him. With his two points of flesh between my fingers, I take control. He doesn't stop me. He has already submitted himself to my "handiwork." He knows that my fingers will bring him to his knees, bring him to surrender.

I roll his tits between my fingers, feeling, pressing their flesh. I delight in the pain and pleasure on his face, his gentle, and not so gentle, moans. He will do anything to convince me to stop but hopes that I won't. I have him; he is mine. Bottoms have submitted, have hoped I'd pinch their tits for a reason. They want the pleasure I can give them.

That "gift" is a joy to a top. We do what we do for the pleasure we inflict. We enjoy, vicariously, the pleasure that our bottoms' tits are producing. We can only sense what's going on, but our senses tell us they're having one hell of a good time. We can tell by the glow on their faces, the sighs in their voices that they are having fun.

I don't know what makes it a turn-on for me. I only know that a major reward to being a top is the knowledge that my bottom is satisfied, and that I can give them that satisfaction with my grandmother's clothespins.

OTHER BOOKS FROM

TOYBAG GUIDES: A Workshop In A Book   *$9.95 each*

Canes and Caning by Janet Hardy

Hot Wax and Temperature Play, by Spectrum

Dungeon Emergencies & Supplies, by Jay Wiseman

BDSM/KINK

The Bullwhip Book
Andrew Conway $11.95

The Compleat Spanker
Lady Green $12.95

Erotic Tickling
Michael Moran $13.95

Family Jewels: A Guide to Male Genital Play and Torment
Hardy Haberman $12.95

Flogging
Joseph W. Bean $12.95

Intimate Invasions: The Ins and Outs of Erotic Enema Play
M.R. Strict $13.95

Jay Wiseman's Erotic Bondage Handbook
Jay Wiseman $16.95

The Loving Dominant
John Warren $16.95

Miss Abernathy's Concise Slave Training Manual
Christina Abernathy $12.95

The Mistress Manual: The Good Girl's Guide to Female Dominance
Mistress Lorelei $16.95

The Sexually Dominant Woman: A Workbook for Nervous Beginners
Lady Green $11.95

SM 101: A Realistic Introduction
Jay Wiseman $24.95

Training With Miss Abernathy: A Workbook for Erotic Slaves and Their Owners
Christina Abernathy $13.95

GENERAL SEXUALITY

Big Big Love: A Sourcebook on Sex for People of Size and Those Who Love Them
Hanne Blank $15.95

*Please include $3 for first book and $1 for each additional book
with your order to cover shipping and handling costs, plus $10 for
overseas orders.*

GREENERY PRESS

The Bride Wore Black Leather... And He Looked Fabulous!: An Etiquette Guide for the Rest of Us
Andrew Campbell $11.95

The Ethical Slut: A Guide to Infinite Sexual Possibilities
Dossie Easton & Catherine A. Liszt $16.95

A Hand in the Bush: The Fine Art of Vaginal Fisting
Deborah Addington $13.95

Health Care Without Shame: A Handbook for the Sexually Diverse and Their Caregivers
Charles Moser, Ph.D., M.D. $11.95

Look Into My Eyes: How to Use Hypnosis to Bring Out the Best in Your Sex Life
Peter Masters $16.95

Phone Sex: Oral Thrills and Aural Skills
Miranda Austin $15.95

Photography for Perverts
Charles Gatewood $27.95

Sex Disasters... And How to Survive Them
Charles Moser, Ph.D., M.D. and Janet W. Hardy $16.95

Tricks... To Please a Man *and* **Tricks... To Please a Woman**
both by Jay Wiseman $14.95 ea.

Turning Pro: A Guide to Sex Work for the Ambitious and the Intrigued
Magdalene Meretrix $16.95

When Someone You Love Is Kinky
Dossie Easton & Catherine A. Liszt $15.95

FICTION

... But I Know What You Want: 25 Sex Tales for the Different
James Williams $13.95

Love, Sal: letters from a boy in The City
Sal Iacopelli, ill. Phil Foglio $13.95

Murder At Roissy
John Warren $15.95

Haughty Spirit
The Warrior Within
The Warrior Enchained
all by Sharon Green $11.95 ea.

VISA/MC accepted. Order from Greenery Press, 3403 Piedmont Ave. #301, Oakland, CA 94611 510/652-2596
www.greenerypress.com.